PREGNANCY BOOK FOR FIRST TIME MOM 2024: CHILDBEARING SIMPLIFIED

Winnie R. Adams

Copyright

© 2024 by Winnie R.Adams

Disclaimer:

This book's contents are provided solely for informational reasons. It is not meant to serve as a replacement for expert medical advice, diagnosis, or care. When in doubt about a medical problem, never hesitate to consult your doctor or another trained healthcare professional. Never ignore medical advice from professionals or put off getting it because of something you've read in this book.

The correctness, application, fitness, and completeness of the information in this book are not warranted or represented by the author or publisher. They make no representations regarding merchantability, fitness for a particular purpose, or implicit or stated guarantees. Never will the writer or publisher be held accountable for any kind of loss or other damages, including but not limited to special, incidental, consequential, or other damages.

The views and opinions expressed in this book are those of the author and do not necessarily reflect the official policy or position of any other individual, agency, organization, or company.

About the author

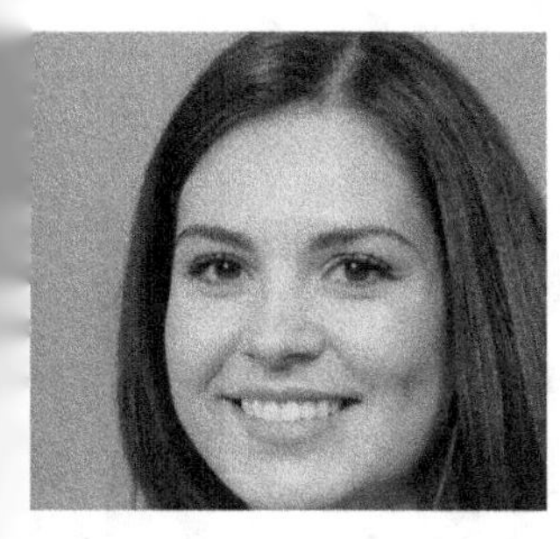

Winnie R. Adams, the author of "Pregnancy book for first time moms 2024: Childbearing Simplified," is a passionate advocate for reproductive health and wellness. With a background in Nutrition, Adams brings a unique blend of expertise, empathy, and a commitment to empowering individuals on their fertility and pregnancy journey.

Having witnessed the challenges that many face in their quest for parenthood, Adams embarked on extensive research, delving into the realms of nutrition, lifestyle, and holistic approaches to fertility.

"Pregnancy book for first time moms 2024" is Winnie's latest endeavor to share her wealth of knowledge with a broader audience. Inspired by her patients' stories and her own experiences as a mother, this book is a culmination of years of expertise and a genuine desire to support women through one of life's most significant experiences. Winnie's approach is holistic, emphasizing the importance of physical, emotional, and mental well-being throughout pregnancy and childbirth.

When she is not writing, Winnie enjoys spending time with her family, practicing yoga, and advocating for maternal health initiatives. Her warm, compassionate approach and dedication to her patients make her a beloved figure in the community and a trusted guide for expectant mothers everywhere.

Winnie Adams believes that every woman deserves a positive and empowering childbirth experience, and she hopes this book will be a valuable resource for women around the world. She is also the Author of book "Optimizing Her Fertility"

TABLE OF CONTENTS

INTRODUCTION

Welcome to the "Pregnancy book for first-time moms 2024"! One of a woman's most fascinating experiences is giving birth to a child. The process of becoming a mother is filled with excitement and joy, but it can also be fraught with fear and uncertainty. This extensive aide means to give hopeful moms the information, viable direction, and backing they need to explore labor effectively.

Important topics like nutrition during pregnancy, coping mechanisms for labor pain, easing labor and delivery exercises, mental preparation, and postpartum recovery are discussed throughout this book. Whether you are a first-time mother or are preparing for a second child, this book will help you make informed decisions, embrace the birthing experience, and embark on the journey of motherhood with strength and resilience.

From understanding the stages of pregnancy to creating a bespoke birth plan, we cover everything you need to know to prepare for a painless and empowering birth. As you leave on this inconceivable excursion of carrying new life into the world, this guide means to facilitate your feelings of trepidation, energize unwinding, and develop a good outlook with viable counsel, master exhortation, and motivating stories.

Let this book be your companion as you embrace the miracle of childbirth and begin the beautiful adventure of motherhood.

PART 1:   Understanding Pregnancy

Chapter1 -Introduction to Pregnancy: Exploring the miraculous journey of pregnancy and the changes a woman's body undergoes.

The beginning of a new life and the expansion of a family are both marked by pregnancy, which is a profound and transformative experience. As a woman's body adapts to support the development of a new human being, this time is marked by significant physiological, emotional, and psychological changes. This journey, which is frequently referred to as miraculous, involves remarkable adaptations and intricate biological processes. In this thorough investigation, we will dive into the phases of pregnancy, the physiological changes a lady's body goes through, and the profound and mental effect of this life changing experience.

The Stages of Pregnancy Typically, there are three trimesters, each lasting about three months, during pregnancy. Both the mother and the developing fetus experience distinct changes and milestones during each trimester.

First Trimester (Weeks 1 through 12) Conception marks the beginning of the first trimester, when a sperm fertilizes an egg and produces a zygote. After fertilization, this zygote divides quickly into a blastocyst, which inserts itself into the uterine wall around the sixth day. This denotes the start of early stage advancement.

Development of the Embryo: The embryo goes through crucial stages of development in the first trimester. It is referred to as a fetus by the eighth week. The significant organs and frameworks start to shape, including the heart, cerebrum, spinal string, and appendages. Because it establishes the foundation for the baby's growth and development, this time is crucial.

Hormonal Changes: The rise in human chorionic gonadotropin (hCG) levels, which can be seen in pregnancy tests, is one of the first signs of pregnancy. Additionally, the body produces more of the essential hormones progesterone and estrogen, which support pregnancy and prevent menstruation.

Physical alterations: During the first trimester, many women experience morning sickness, or fatigue, nausea, and vomiting. Hormonal changes are frequently to blame for these symptoms. Breast tenderness, frequent urination, and mood swings are additional changes.

Second Trimester (Weeks 13–26) The second trimester of a pregnancy is frequently regarded as the most peaceful time. Numerous early side effects, like morning disorder, start to die down, and the gamble of unsuccessful labor diminishes essentially.

Growth of the Fetus: The fetus's rapid growth continues. It has developed fingerprints, is able to hear sounds, and continues to develop its organs by the end of the second trimester. Quickening is when the fetus begins to move, and the mother can feel these movements.

Physical alterations: As the uterus expands, the belly becomes more prominent. Women might notice a "baby bump" and start to feel the baby moving. The skin may change, such as the appearance of a dark line (linea nigra) that runs from the belly button to the pubic area and darkens the nipples. As the skin stretches, it may also develop stretch marks.

Nutrition and Wellness: It is essential to eat a well-balanced diet high in essential nutrients like calcium, iron, and folic acid during this time. The baby's development and any potential issues are monitored during regular prenatal exams.

The third trimester, which lasts from weeks 27 to 40, is the final stage of pregnancy before the baby is born. The body keeps on planning for work and conveyance, and the embryo goes through conclusive development and development.

Growth of the Fetus: The fetus develops its organs, particularly the lungs, and rapidly increases its weight in preparation for birth. The fetus typically settles into a head-down position in the pelvis by the end of the third trimester, signaling readiness for delivery.

Physical alterations: The mother may experience increased discomfort as the baby grows, such as back pain, ankle and foot swelling, and shortness of breath. As the body prepares for labor, false labor pains known as Braxton Hicks contraction may occur.

Groundwork for Birth: In preparation fo childbirth, the body makes relaxin, a hormone tha helps soften the cervix and relax the pelvi ligaments. The first form of breast milk, colostrum may begin to leak from the breasts.

Physiological Changes During Pregnancy

Pregnancy sets off a huge number of physiologica changes in a lady's body, intended to help the developing baby and set up the mother for labo and breastfeeding. Nearly every organ system i affected by these changes.

Cardiovascular Framework

The cardiovascular framework goes through huge changes in accordance with oblige the expanded requests of pregnancy. During the second trimester, blood volume rises by 30 to 50 percent. This increment upholds the developing baby and placenta and makes up for blood misfortune during conveyance. In addition, the heart rate rises, and he heart slightly expands to accommodate the ncreased blood flow.

The Respiratory System Pregnancy has a number of effects on the respiratory system. The diaphragm is pressed against the growing uterus, reducing lung capacity and frequently resulting in shortness of breath. Progesterone increases tidal volume and respiratory rate, ensuring that both the mother and the fetus receive enough oxygen.

Renal Framework

The kidneys work harder during pregnancy to channel expanded blood volume and discharge byproducts from both the mother and the embryo. This frequently leads to more frequent urination and increased urine production. Pregnant women may be more likely to get urinary tract infections because the renal pelvis and ureters may dilate.

The Digestive Tract Hormonal changes, particularly elevated levels of progesterone, relax the gastrointestinal tract's smooth muscles, stymieing digestion and frequently resulting in constipation. Heartburn or acid reflux can be brought on by the relaxation of the lower esophageal sphincter. These symptoms are made worse by the stomach and intestines being displaced by the growing uterus.

The Endocrine System The endocrine system is very important during pregnancy. As an endocrine organ, the placenta makes hormones like hCG, progesterone, and estrogen. The thyroid gland expands and produces more hormone, which is necessary for the metabolism and development of the fetal brain. The pancreas adjusts by expanding insulin creation to control blood glucose levels, yet in certain ladies, this variation comes up short, prompting gestational diabetes.

The Musculoskeletal System, the Musculoskeletal System goes through a number of changes to accommodate the growing fetus and get ready for giving birth. In order to facilitate childbirth, the hormone relaxin softens the ligaments and joints, particularly in the pelvis. Instability and joint pain can result from this. Changes in posture and lower back pain are requently brought on by the uterus expanding, which shifts the center of gravity.

Integumentary Framework
The skin and related structures go through different changes during pregnancy. Hormonal changes can cause hyperpigmentation, such as the appearance of the linea nigra and darkened nipples, while increased blood flow can produce a healthy glow. The stretching of the skin can lead to stretch marks, or striae gravidarum.

Changes in Emotion and Mental State In addition to the physical changes, pregnancy brings about significant changes in mental and emotional state. Hormonal changes, physical discomfort, and the anticipation of having children all play a role in these shifts.

Emotional Responses Pregnancy frequently elicits a variety of feelings, ranging from excitement and joy to anxiety and fear. Mood swings, heightened sensitivity, and emotional vulnerability may result from the hormonal changes. The feelings of attachment and bonding with the unborn child rise in many women.

Mental Changes

Eager moms frequently go through a mental change as they get ready for their new job. Accepting the reality of the pregnancy, getting ready for the arrival of the baby, and developing a maternal identity are all parts of this process, which is also referred to as "maternal adaptation." Personal beliefs, social support, and previous experiences all play a role in this adjustment.

Mental health considerations While pregnancy can be a joyful time for many, it can also present challenges to mental health. Pregnancy-related depression and anxiety can affect a woman's well-being and the health of her unborn child. If pregnant women experience persistent feelings of sadness, anxiety, or distress, it is essential for them to seek assistance from support groups, mental health professionals, and healthcare providers.

The Function of Prenatal Care Prenatal care is necessary for identifying and managing potential omplications, providing education and support, and keeping an eye on the health of the mother and the fetus. Typical routines for prenatal visits include:

Exams of the body: assessing the fetus's growth and development as well as weight gain and blood pressure.

Tests in the lab: Evaluating for conditions like gestational diabetes, frailty, and diseases.

Scans by Ultrasound: Keeping an eye on the position and development of the fetus.

Counseling and education: distributing information regarding nutrition, exercise, preparation for childbirth, and breastfeeding.

Additionally, discussions about birth plans, pain management options, and postpartum care are part of prenatal care. It is a basic part of guaranteeing a solid pregnancy and a positive labor insight.

Preparing for Childbirth As the due date gets closer, pregnant women and their partners need to get ready for the birth of their child. There are several important aspects to this preparation:

Labor Instruction Classes

Labor instruction classes give significant data about the work and conveyance process, tormen the board choices, and post pregnancy care. These classes may assist new parents in developing sense of self-assurance and preparing for the birth experience.

Birth Plan Pregnant women can tell their healthcare team about their preferences for labor and delivery when they make a birth plan. Preferences for pain management, the presence o support people, and interventions like episiotomy or cesarean section are all examples of this. Having a plan can help ensure that the mother's wishes are taken into consideration during childbirth, despite the fact that flexibility is crucial.

Support System During pregnancy and childbirth, having a solid support system is essential. A partner, friends, family, and medical professionals are all examples of this. During labor and delivery, support individuals can offer emotional encouragement, practical assistance, and advocacy.

Post pregnancy Arranging

Making arrangements for the post pregnancy time frame is additionally significant. This includes learning about the signs of postpartum depression, getting help at home, and preparing for breastfeeding. Having a plan in place can support the mother's recovery and ease the transition to parenthood.

The Marvel of Life

Pregnancy is many times depicted as a marvelous excursion since it includes the creation and improvement of another life. The process is characterized by extraordinary biological and emotional changes from conception to birth. The body undergoes remarkable adaptations to support the fetus's growth and development at each stage of pregnancy, which brings with it new developments and milestones.

Moments of profound connection and wonder include the sensation of a baby's first movement, hearing its heartbeat, and seeing its image on an ultrasound. Pregnancy likewise brings a more profound comprehension of the body's capacities and the strength and flexibility of ladies.

Chapter 2 Stages of Pregnancy

Detailing the trimesters and what to expect during each phase.

Common Discomforts: Addressing common pregnancy discomforts and offering tips for relief.

Pregnancy is a remarkable journey divided int three trimesters, each approximately three month long. Each trimester comes with its own set c developments, changes, and expectations for bot the mother and the developing fetu Understanding what to expect during eac trimester can help prepare expectant mothers fo the physical, emotional, and psychological change that accompany pregnancy.

First Trimester (Weeks 1-12)

The first trimester marks the beginning o pregnancy, starting from the first day of the las menstrual period (LMP) to the end of week 12 This phase is critical for the development of the embryo and the establishment of the pregnancy.

Developmental Milestones

- **Weeks 1-4:** Conception occurs, and the fertilized egg (zygote) undergoes rapid cell division to form a blastocyst, which implants into the uterine lining. This marks the beginning of the embryonic stage.

- **Weeks 5-8:** The embryo's major organs and systems start to form. The heart begins to beat, and structures such as the brain, spinal cord, and limbs start to develop.
- **Weeks 9-12:** The embryo transitions into a fetus. By the end of the first trimester, the fetus has developed most of its organs, although they are still maturing. Facial features, fingers, and toes become more distinct.

Physical Changes

- **Hormonal Fluctuations:** The body produces high levels of hormones such as human chorionic gonadotropin (hCG), progesterone, and estrogen to support the pregnancy. These hormonal changes can lead to common symptoms like nausea, vomiting (morning sickness), fatigue, and breast tenderness.
- **Weight Gain:** Some women may experience slight weight gain, although significant weight gain is more common in the second and third trimesters.

- **Frequent Urination:** Increased blood flow to the pelvic area and hormonal changes can cause frequent urination.
- **Mood Swings:** Hormonal fluctuations can also lead to mood swings, irritability, and emotional sensitivity.

Common Concerns and Tips

- **Morning Sickness:** Eating small, frequent meals and avoiding strong odors or foods that trigger nausea can help manage morning sickness. Ginger and vitamin B6 supplements can provide relief from these symptoms.
- **Fatigue:** Resting and maintaining a healthy diet can help combat fatigue. Regular light exercise, such as walking, can also boost energy levels.
- **Prenatal Care:** The first prenatal visit typically occurs around week 8. This visit includes a thorough medical history, physical examination, and necessary tests such as blood work and an ultrasound to confirm the pregnancy and check for a fetal heartbeat.

Second Trimester (Weeks 13-26)

The second trimester is considered the most comfortable phase of pregnancy by most women. Many early symptoms, such as nausea and fatigue, begin to subside, and the risk of miscarriage decreases significantly.

Developmental Milestones

- **Weeks 13-16:** The fetus continues to grow rapidly. The skeleton begins to harden from cartilage to bone, and the reproductive organs become more developed.
- **Weeks 17-20:** The fetus can hear sounds, and its movements become more coordinated. By week 20, the mother may start to feel fetal movements, known as quickening.
- **Weeks 21-26:** The fetus's skin becomes less translucent, and fat begins to develop under the skin. The fetus's lungs produce surfactant, a substance that helps the lungs function after birth.

Physical Changes

- **Growing Belly:** The uterus expands, and the belly becomes more pronounced. Most women start to show a noticeable baby bump around this time.
- **Skin Changes:** Hormonal changes can cause the skin to darken, resulting in the appearance of the linea nigra (a dark line running from the belly button to the pubic area) and darkening of the nipples. Stretch marks may also develop.
- **Breast Changes:** The breasts continue to grow in preparation for breastfeeding, and some women may notice colostrum (early breast milk) leaking from their nipples.
- **Increased Energy:** Many women experience a boost in energy levels and an improvement in mood as early symptoms wane.

Common Concerns and Tips

- **Back Pain:** As the belly grows, the center of gravity shifts, which can lead to back pain. Practicing good posture, wearing supportive shoes, and engaging in prenatal yoga or gentle stretching exercises can help alleviate discomfort.

- **Heartburn and Indigestion:** Hormonal changes relax the muscles of the digestive tract, which can cause heartburn. Eating smaller meals, avoiding spicy and fatty foods, and not lying down immediately after eating can help manage these symptoms.
- **Prenatal Visits:** Regular prenatal visits continue to monitor the baby's growth and development. Anomaly scans, such as the mid-pregnancy ultrasound around 20 weeks, check for any structural abnormalities in the fetus.

Third Trimester (Weeks 27-40)

The third trimester is the final phase of pregnancy, that precedes the birth of the baby. The body undergoes final preparations for labor and delivery, and the fetus undergoes significant growth and maturation.

Developmental Milestones

- **Weeks 27-30:** The fetus's brain continues to develop rapidly, and the nervous system matures. The fetus starts to gain more weight and develop a layer of fat under the skin.
- **Weeks 31-34:** The fetus's bones fully develop, although they remain soft and pliable for birth. The fetus's eyes can open and close, and it can detect light changes.
- **Weeks 35-40:** The fetus moves into a head-down position in the pelvis in preparation for birth. The lungs mature, and the fetus continues to gain weight and store nutrients such as iron and calcium.

Physical Changes

- **Increased Belly Size:** The belly grows larger, and the uterus can be felt near the rib cage. This can cause discomfort and difficulty breathing as the uterus pushes against the diaphragm.
- **Braxton Hicks Contractions:** These are irregular, painless contractions that help prepare the uterus for labor. They are

different from true labor contractions, which are regular and progressively stronger.

- **Swelling:** Swelling of the ankles, feet, and hands is common due to increased fluid retention and pressure from the growing uterus.
- **Fatigue and Discomfort:** Many women experience increased fatigue, back pain, and difficulty sleeping due to the size and weight of the baby.

Common Concerns and Tips

- **Labor Signs:** Understanding the signs of labor, such as regular contractions, water breaking, and the passage of the mucus plug, can help prepare for the onset of labor. Attending childbirth education classes can provide valuable information and confidence for labor and delivery.
- **Preterm Labor:** Recognizing the signs of preterm labor, such as regular contractions before 37 weeks, pelvic pressure, and changes in vaginal discharge, is important. Contacting a healthcare provider

immediately if these signs occur can help manage and prevent preterm birth.

- **Prenatal Visits:** More frequent prenatal visits occur during the third trimester to closely monitor the baby's position, growth, and overall health. Discussing the birth plan, pain management options, and any concerns with the healthcare provider is essential during these visits.

PART 2: The Importance of Nutrition During Pregnancy for a Smooth Labor and Delivery

Chapter 3 Understanding Nutritional Needs

Exploring the essential nutrients needed during pregnancy for the health of both mother and baby.

Planning a Balanced Diet: Providing guidance on creating a nutritious meal plan that supports the development of the baby and helps alleviate common pregnancy discomforts.

As a time of profound physiological change pregnancy necessitates increased nutritional requirements to support mother and baby's health Nutritional support during pregnancy can help alleviate common pregnancy discomforts and ensure the best possible fetal development Understanding the fundamental supplements expected during this period is essential for making a fair and nutritious eating routine.

During Pregnancy, Essential Nutrients Folic Acid (Folate):

Importance: Folic acid is essential for preventing spina bifida and other neural tube defects (NTDs). It assumes a significant part in DNA union and cell division.

Sources: Verdant green vegetables, citrus organic products, beans, peas, lentils, and strengthened grains.

Suggested Admission: 600-800 micrograms everyday.

ron:

mportance: Iron is needed to make hemoglobin, which carries oxygen throughout the blood. Expanded blood volume during pregnancy requires more iron to guarantee satisfactory oxygen supply to both mother and child.

Sources: Vegetables, fish, red meat, lentils, beans, spinach, and cereals with added iron

The Recommended Dose: daily of 27 milligrams.

Calcium:

Importance: The development of the baby's bones, teeth, heart, nerves, and muscles all depend on calcium. Additionally, it aids in preventing maternal bone loss.

Sources: Fortified plant-based milk, dairy products like milk, cheese, and yogurt, as well as leafy greens, almonds, and tofu.

The Recommended Dose: daily of 1,00(milligrams.

D vitamin:

Importance: Vitamin D guides in the retention of calcium and is fundamental for bone wellbeing and safe capability.

Sources: Fortified milk, fatty fish like salmon and sardines, eggs, and sunlight are all beneficial.

The Recommended Dose: 600-800 IU per day

DHA and EPA, or omega-3 fatty acids, are

Importance: Omega-3 fatty acids are necessary for the brain and eyes of the baby to develop. Additionally, they aid in maternal heart health.

Sources: Omega-3-enriched eggs, flaxseeds, chia seeds, walnuts, and fatty fish like salmon, mackerel, and trout

The Recommended Dose: 200-300 mg of DHA per day.

Protein:

Importance: The development of fetal tissues and the placenta are both dependent on protein for their growth and repair.

Sources: Lean meats, poultry, fish, eggs, dairy, legumes, nuts, seeds, and soy products are all good sources of protein.

The Recommended Dose: Around 75-100 grams day to day, contingent upon individual requirements.

C vitamin:

Importance: Vitamin C helps the body absorb iron better, boosts the immune system, and makes connective tissue and collagen grow.

Sources: Citrus organic products (oranges, grapefruits, lemons), strawberries, ringer peppers, broccoli, and tomatoes.

The Recommended Dose: 85 micrograms per day.

Fiber:

Importance: Fiber forestalls stoppage, a typical issue during pregnancy because of hormonal changes and the strain of the developing uterus on the digestion tracts.

Sources: legumes, nuts, seeds, whole grains, and vegetables

The Recommended Dose: 25-30 grams everyday.

Creating a Healthy Meal Plan During pregnancy, incorporating a variety of foods to ensure adequate intake of essential nutrients is an important part of creating a healthy meal plan. A well-balanced diet can support the development of the fetus, improve the health of the mother, and alleviate common discomforts associated with pregnancy.

Putting together a meal plan for breakfast:

xemplary Meal: Poached egg on whole-grain ast, fortified cereal with milk in a bowl, and range juice in a glass

ourishing Advantages: For a good start to the ay, this meal contains vitamin C, protein, iron, ber, and healthy fats.

nack at Midday:

nack Example: Greek yogurt topped with a few erries and some chia seeds.

Vholesome Advantages: Omega-3 fatty acids, alcium, protein, and antioxidants all in one.

unch:

Exemplary Meal: Mixed greens, cucumber, bell peppers, quinoa, and a lemon-tahini dressing make up this grilled chicken salad.

Benefits for the diet: This meal has a good balance of carbohydrates and healthy fats, and it is full of protein, vitamins, minerals, and fiber.

Lunchtime Snack:

Snack Example: Almond butter and apple slices, c
a handful of nuts and dried fruit.

Nourishing Advantages: contains essentia
vitamins and minerals, protein, healthy fats, an
fiber.

Dinner:

Exemplary Meal: roasted sweet potatoes and
steamed broccoli served alongside baked salmon.

Benefits for the diet: Omega-3 fatty acids, protein
fiber, vitamins, and minerals in this meal aid in
fetal development and overall health.

Dinner Snack:

Snack Example: a smoothie made with spinach,
banana, and fortified plant-based milk or a small
bowl of cottage cheese with pineapple chunks.

Benefits for the diet: combines protein, calcium, vitamins, and minerals to provide a balanced meal at the end of the day.

Variety is the Key to a Healthy Pregnancy Diet:

Consuming a variety of foods ensures that you get all of the nutrients you need. Incorporate various varieties and kinds of foods grown from the ground, entire grains, lean proteins, and solid fats in your eating regimen.

Keep hydrated:

To stay hydrated throughout the day, drink a lot of water. At least 8-10 glasses of water everyday. Amniotic fluid levels can be maintained and overall health can be supported by hydration.

Control portions:

You do not have to eat twice as much to feed two people. Instead of significantly increasing calories, focus on foods that are high in nutrients. Pay attention to your body's craving and completion prompts.

Eat less processed food:

Decrease the admission of handled food varieties, sweet tidbits, and drinks. These items frequently have few nutrients and a lot of empty calories.

Use caution when adding:

Vitamins for pregnant women can help with missing nutrients, but they should not take the place of a healthy diet. Counsel your medical services supplier prior to beginning any enhancements to guarantee they meet your singular necessities.

Careful Eating:

By paying attention to your food choices and savoring each bite, you can practice mindful eating. This can aid in digestion and prevent overeating.

Address Common Gripes:

For vomiting: Avoid greasy or sour foods and eat small, frequent meals.

For bloating: Keep hydrated and eat more fiber.

For indigestion: Eat more modest dinners all the more oftentimes, stay away from hot and acidic food sources, and abstain from resting following eating.

Chapter 4 Managing Pregnancy-related Conditions Addressing specific dietary considerations for conditions such as gestational diabetes, preeclampsia, and morning sickness.

Foods to Support Labor: Discussing foods rich in nutrients such as omega-3 fatty acids, protein, and iron that can help prepare the body for childbirth.

Hydration: Emphasizing the importance of staying hydrated during pregnancy and labor, and providing tips for increasing fluid intake.

Snacks for Energy: Offering healthy snack ideas to maintain energy levels during labor and delivery.

Pregnancy can sometimes bring about certain health conditions that require specific dietary management. Proper nutrition is crucial not only for the health of the baby but also for managing these conditions effectively. This guide will cover dietary considerations for gestational diabetes, preeclampsia, and morning sickness, offering practical tips to help expectant mothers navigate these challenges.

Gestational Diabetes

Gestational diabetes (GDM) is a condition where blood sugar levels become elevated during pregnancy. Managing gestational diabetes primarily involves dietary adjustments to maintain stable blood glucose levels.

Dietary Considerations

1. **Carbohydrate Management:**
   - **Balanced Carbohydrate Intake:** Focus on complex carbohydrates that are high in fiber and have a lower glycemic index. These include whole

grains, legumes, vegetables, and som fruits.

- **Portion Control:** Distribut carbohydrate intake evenl throughout the day to avoid spikes i blood sugar levels. This means havin smaller, more frequent meals an snacks.
- **Carbohydrate Counting** Monitoring and controllin carbohydrate intake can help manage blood glucose levels effectively.

2. **Protein and Fat:**

- **Lean Proteins:** Incorporate lear sources of protein such as chicken, turkey, fish, eggs, tofu, and legumes. Protein helps stabilize blood sugar levels.
- **Healthy Fats:** Include healthy fats from sources like avocados, nuts, seeds, and olive oil. These fats can provide satiety and help with blood sugar control.

3. **Fiber:**

- o **High-Fiber Foods:** Foods high in fiber, such as vegetables, fruits with skin, whole grains, and legumes, help slow the absorption of glucose and improve blood sugar control.

4. **Meal Timing and Frequency:**
   - o **Regular Meals:** Eating regular, balanced meals and snacks can help maintain consistent blood sugar levels. Avoid long gaps between meals.
   - o **Morning Meal:** A protein-rich breakfast can help prevent morning blood sugar spikes.

5. **Monitoring Blood Sugar Levels:**
   - o **Frequent Monitoring:** Regularly checking blood glucose levels as recommended by a healthcare provider can help manage gestational diabetes effectively.

Sample Meal Plan for Gestational Diabetes

- **Breakfast:** Scrambled eggs with spinach and whole-grain toast.

- **Mid-Morning Snack:** Greek yogurt with a handful of berries.
- **Lunch:** Grilled chicken salad with mixed greens, quinoa, and a lemon vinaigrette.
- **Afternoon Snack:** Apple slices with almond butter.
- **Dinner:** Baked salmon with roasted sweet potatoes and steamed broccoli.
- **Evening Snack:** A small bowl of cottage cheese with pineapple chunks.

Preeclampsia

Preeclampsia is a pregnancy complication characterized by high blood pressure and potential damage to other organs, most often the liver and kidneys. Dietary management can play a role in controlling blood pressure and supporting overall health.

Dietary Considerations

1. **Sodium Intake:**
   - **Limit Sodium:** Reducing sodium intake can help manage blood pressure. Avoid processed foods,

canned soups, and high-sodium snacks. Opt for fresh, whole foods.

- o **Flavor with Herbs:** Use herbs and spices to flavor food instead of salt.

2. **Hydration:**
   - o **Adequate Hydration:** Drinking plenty of water helps maintain healthy blood pressure and supports kidney function.

3. **Calcium:**
   - o **Calcium-Rich Foods:** Consuming calcium-rich foods such as dairy products, leafy greens, and fortified plant-based milks can support vascular health and blood pressure control.

4. **Potassium:**
   - o **Potassium-Rich Foods:** Potassium helps balance sodium levels in the body and supports healthy blood pressure. Include bananas, sweet potatoes, spinach, and avocados in your diet.

5. **Antioxidants:**

- ○ **Antioxidant-Rich Foods:** Foods high in antioxidants, such as berries, nuts and green leafy vegetables, can help reduce oxidative stress and inflammation associated with preeclampsia.

Sample Meal Plan for Preeclampsia

- **Breakfast:** Oatmeal with sliced bananas, chia seeds, and a splash of almond milk.
- **Mid-Morning Snack:** Carrot sticks with hummus.
- **Lunch:** Quinoa bowl with mixed greens, cherry tomatoes, cucumber, chickpeas, and a tahini dressing.
- **Afternoon Snack:** A handful of unsalted nuts and a small apple.
- **Dinner:** Grilled chicken with sautéed spinach and roasted sweet potatoes.
- **Evening Snack:** A small bowl of mixed berries.

Morning Sickness

Morning sickness, characterized by nausea and vomiting, is common during the first trimester of pregnancy. Dietary adjustments can help manage symptoms and ensure adequate nutrition.

Dietary Considerations

1. **Small, Frequent Meals:**
   - **Avoid Large Meals:** Eating smaller, more frequent meals can help prevent nausea. Large meals can overwhelm the digestive system and exacerbate symptoms.
   - **Frequent Snacking:** Having healthy snacks available can help maintain blood sugar levels and reduce nausea.
2. **Ginger:**
   - **Ginger Remedies:** Ginger has natural anti-nausea properties. Try ginger tea, ginger ale, ginger candies, or adding fresh ginger to meals.
3. **Bland Foods:**
   - **Bland, Easy-to-Digest Foods:** Foods such as crackers, toast, rice, and applesauce can be easier to tolerate.

Avoid spicy, fatty, or overly seasone foods.

4. **Cold Foods:**
   - **Cold or Room-Temperature Foods** Cold foods can sometimes be mor tolerable than hot foods, which ma have stronger smells that trigge nausea.

5. **Hydration:**
   - **Stay Hydrated:** Sip on water, clea broths, or herbal teas throughout th day. Ice chips and popsicles can als help maintain hydration.

6. **Avoid Triggers:**
   - **Identify and Avoid Triggers:** Certain smells, foods, or environments can trigger nausea. Identifying and avoiding these triggers can help manage symptoms.

Sample Meal Plan for Morning Sickness

- **Breakfast:** Plain toast with a light spread of almond butter and a small banana.
- **Mid-Morning Snack:** A handful of crackers with a slice of mild cheese.

- **Lunch:** Chicken broth with rice and steamed carrots.
- **Afternoon Snack:** A small bowl of applesauce.
- **Dinner:** Baked potato with a small amount of sour cream and steamed green beans.
- **Evening Snack:** Ginger tea and a small bowl of plain popcorn.

Managing pregnancy-related conditions such as gestational diabetes, preeclampsia, and morning sickness requires specific dietary considerations to ensure the health and well-being of both mother and baby. A balanced and nutritious diet tailored to the individual needs of each condition can help alleviate symptoms and support a healthy pregnancy. Consulting with a healthcare provider or a registered dietitian can provide personalized guidance and support throughout this journey.

PART 3: Exercise and Movement During Pregnancy

Chapter 5 Benefits of Exercise: Exploring the physical and mental benefits of staying active during pregnancy, including improved stamina, mood, and easier labor.

Safe Exercises: Providing a range of safe exercises suitable for pregnant women, including prenatal yoga, swimming, and walking.

Staying active during pregnancy offers a multitude of benefits, both physical and mental, for expectant mothers. Engaging in regular exercise can improve stamina, enhance mood, and contribute to smoother labor and delivery process. Understanding these benefits can motivate pregnant women to incorporate appropriate physical activities into their daily routines ensuring a healthier and more enjoyable pregnancy journey.

Physical Benefits of Exercise During Pregnancy

1. **Improved Stamina and Endurance:**
   - **Increased Energy Levels:** Regular exercise helps boost energy by improving cardiovascular health and increasing blood flow. This can counteract pregnancy-related fatigue and provide more vitality throughout the day.
   - **Enhanced Endurance:** Building stamina through activities such as walking, swimming, or prenatal yoga prepares the body for the demands of labor. Endurance training helps

muscles function more efficiently, which is beneficial during the prolonged physical effort of childbirth.

2. **Better Weight Management:**
   - **Healthy Weight Gain:** Exercise helps regulate weight gain by burning excess calories and maintaining muscle mass. This can reduce the risk of gestational diabetes and preeclampsia, conditions often associated with excessive weight gain during pregnancy.
   - **Easier Postpartum Recovery:** Maintaining a healthy weight during pregnancy can facilitate quicker postpartum recovery, making it easier to return to pre-pregnancy fitness levels.

3. **Reduced Pregnancy Discomforts:**
   - **Alleviated Back Pain:** Strengthening the core muscles through exercise can help reduce back pain, a common complaint during pregnancy. Activities like swimming and prenatal

Pilates target the back and abdomina muscles, providing relief.

- o **Decreased Swelling:** Regula physical activity improves circulation, which can help reduce swelling in the legs, ankles, and feet by preventing fluid retention.
- o **Eased Constipation:** Exercise stimulates intestinal function, helping to prevent constipation, another common issue during pregnancy.

4. **Preparation for Labor:**

- o **Stronger Muscles:** Exercise strengthens muscles used during labor and delivery, such as the pelvic floor, which plays a crucial role in childbirth. Strengthening these muscles can lead to more efficient contractions and potentially shorter labor.
- o **Increased Flexibility:** Prenatal yoga and stretching exercises enhance flexibility, which can aid in accommodating the physical demands of labor and delivery. Improved

flexibility also helps with different labor positions and can make the birthing process more comfortable.

Mental Benefits of Exercise During Pregnancy

1. **Enhanced Mood and Emotional Well-being:**
   - **Reduced Stress and Anxiety:** Exercise releases endorphins, the body's natural stress relievers, which help reduce anxiety and promote a sense of well-being. Physical activity can also lower levels of cortisol, the stress hormone.
   - **Improved Sleep:** Regular exercise promotes better sleep patterns, which can be disrupted during pregnancy due to physical discomfort and hormonal changes. Better sleep contributes to improved mood and overall mental health.
   - **Decreased Risk of Depression:** Staying active during pregnancy can lower the risk of prenatal and postpartum depression. Exercise

provides a natural outlet for stress and negative emotions, contributing to a more positive outlook.

2. **Increased Self-Esteem and Body Image:**
   - **Positive Body Image:** Exercise helps pregnant women feel more in control of their changing bodies, promoting a positive body image. Staying active can improve confidence and self-esteem, which are crucial during the emotional journey of pregnancy.
   - **Sense of Accomplishment:** Setting and achieving fitness goals, even small ones, can provide a sense of accomplishment and empowerment, enhancing overall emotional well-being.

3. **Better Social Connections:**
   - **Community and Support:** Participating in group fitness classes, such as prenatal yoga or swimming, can foster a sense of community and provide emotional support. Sharing experiences with other expectant

mothers can alleviate feelings of isolation and build a support network.

Safe Exercise Guidelines for Pregnancy

While the benefits of exercise during pregnancy are substantial, it is essential to follow safe exercise guidelines to protect both mother and baby.

1. **Consult with a Healthcare Provider:**
   - **Medical Clearance:** Before starting any exercise regimen, it is crucial to consult with a healthcare provider to ensure that physical activity is safe, especially if there are any underlying health conditions or pregnancy complications.
2. **Choose Appropriate Activities:**
   - **Low-Impact Exercises:** Opt for low-impact activities such as walking, swimming, stationary cycling, and prenatal yoga, which are gentle on the joints and reduce the risk of injury.
   - **Avoid High-Risk Activities:** Avoid activities with a high risk of falling or

abdominal trauma, such as contac
sports, skiing, or horseback riding.

3. **Modify Exercises as Needed:**
   o **Adapt to Changes:** As pregnanc
   progresses, modify exercises t
   accommodate the growing belly an
   changing center of gravity. Use prop
   like chairs or walls for support durin;
   balance exercises.

   o **Pay attention to body signals:** Pa;
   attention to your body's signals and
   do not overstretch yourself. Res
   when needed and stay hydrated.

4. **Focus on Core and Pelvic Floor Strength:**
   o **Targeted Exercises:** Incorporate
   exercises that strengthen the core and
   pelvic floor muscles, such as pelvic
   tilts, Kegels, and prenatal Pilates.
   These muscles support the growing
   uterus and prepare for labor.

5. **Stay Hydrated and Avoid Overheating:**
   o **Hydration:** Drink plenty of water
   before, during, and after exercise to
   stay hydrated.

- **Cool Environment:** Exercise in a cool, well-ventilated environment and avoid activities that raise body temperature excessively.

The physical and mental benefits of staying active during pregnancy are profound. Regular exercise can improve stamina, enhance mood, and prepare the body for labor and delivery, contributing to a healthier and more enjoyable pregnancy experience. By following safe exercise guidelines and choosing appropriate activities, expectant mothers can harness the benefits of physical activity, promoting the well-being of both themselves and their babies. Embracing an active lifestyle during pregnancy not only supports immediate health but also lays the foundation for a healthier postpartum recovery and long-term well-being.

Chapter 6 Pelvic Floor Exercises: Detailing the importance of pelvic floor exercises in preparing for childbirth and preventing postpartum complications.

Labor-Preparation Exercises: Introducing exercises specifically designed to prepare the body for the physical demands of labor, such as squats, pelvic tilts, and deep breathing techniques.

Partner-Assisted Techniques: Discussing exercises that partners can assist with to provide support and promote relaxation during labor.

Incorporating Exercise into Daily Routine: Offering practical tips for integrating exercise into daily life during pregnancy, even for those with busy schedules.

Breathing Exercises: Teaching various breathing techniques to promote relaxation, manage pain, and enhance oxygen flow during labor.

elvic floor exercises, often referred to as Kegel exercises, play a crucial role in preparing for childbirth and preventing postpartum complications. These exercises target the pelvic floor muscles, which support the bladder, bowel, and uterus. Strengthening these muscles can lead to a smoother labor, faster postpartum recovery, and a reduction in common pregnancy and postpartum issues such as incontinence and pelvic organ prolapse.

Understanding the Pelvic Floor

The pelvic floor is a group of muscles and ligaments that form a sling across the pelvic cavity. These muscles provide support for the pelvic organs, assist in controlling bladder and bowel movements, and play a significant role in sexual function. During pregnancy, the growing baby places increased pressure on the pelvic floor, potentially weakening these muscles.

Importance of Pelvic Floor Exercises During Pregnancy

1. **Preparation for Childbirth:**

- **Enhanced Muscle Control:** Strong pelvic floor muscles provide better control during labor, helping to manage contractions and facilitate the birthing process. These muscles work actively during the pushing phase of labor.
- **Reduced Risk of Perineal Tearing:** Strengthening and learning to relax the pelvic floor muscles can help reduce the risk of perineal tearing or the need for an episiotomy during childbirth. Better muscle control allows for a more gradual and controlled delivery of the baby.

2. **Prevention of Incontinence:**
   - **Urinary Incontinence:** Pregnancy can increase the risk of urinary incontinence due to the added pressure on the bladder and weakened pelvic floor muscles. Regular pelvic floor exercises help maintain bladder control by strengthening the muscles that support the urethra.

- **Fecal Incontinence:** Strengthening the pelvic floor also helps prevent fecal incontinence by supporting the rectum and maintaining control over bowel movements.

3. **Support for Pelvic Organs:**
   - **Prevention of Pelvic Organ Prolapse:** The pressure from the growing uterus can lead to pelvic organ prolapse, where organs such as the bladder, uterus, or rectum descend into the vaginal canal. Pelvic floor exercises help support these organs, reducing the risk of prolapse during and after pregnancy.

4. **Improved Posture and Reduced Back Pain:**
   - **Postural Support:** Strong pelvic floor muscles contribute to better posture by supporting the spine and pelvic alignment. This can help alleviate common pregnancy-related back pain.

Importance of Pelvic Floor Exercise Postpartum

1. **Faster Recovery:**
   - **Postpartum Healing:** Pelvic floor exercises promote blood flow to the perineum and vaginal area, which aids in the healing process after childbirth. This can speed up recovery and reduce discomfort from perineal tears or episiotomies.
   - **Regaining Muscle Tone:** Regular pelvic floor exercises help restore muscle tone and strength, which may be weakened or stretched during childbirth.
2. **Continued Prevention of Incontinence and Prolapse:**
   - **Long-Term Pelvic Health:** Continuing pelvic floor exercises postpartum helps maintain bladder and bowel control, preventing long-term issues such as urinary and fecal incontinence.

- **Sustained Organ Support:** These exercises provide ongoing support for pelvic organs, reducing the risk of prolapse in the long term.

3. **Enhanced Sexual Health:**
   - **Improved Sensation:** Strong pelvic floor muscles can enhance sexual sensation and satisfaction by increasing blood flow and muscle control in the vaginal area.
   - **Reduced Pain:** Pelvic floor exercises can help reduce postpartum sexual discomfort by promoting muscle relaxation and flexibility.

How to Perform Pelvic Floor Exercises

1. **Identifying the Pelvic Floor Muscles:**
   - **Muscle Awareness:** To identify the pelvic floor muscles, try stopping the flow of urine midstream. The muscles used to do this are the pelvic floor muscles. However, avoid making this a regular exercise as it can lead to incomplete emptying of the bladder.

2. **Basic Kegel Exercise:**

- **Step-by-Step Guide:**
    1. **Find a Comfortable Position:** Sit, stand, or lie down with your knees slightly apart.
    2. **Contract the Muscles:** Tighten the pelvic floor muscles as if you are trying to stop the flow of urine or prevent passing gas.
    3. **Hold the Contraction:** Hold the contraction for 5-10 seconds while breathing normally.
    4. **Relax:** Relax the muscles completely for 5-10 seconds.
    5. **Repeat:** Do this 12-15 times, three times a day.

3. **Incorporating Pelvic Floor Exercises into Daily Life:**
    - **Consistency:** Consistency is key to seeing benefits. Try to incorporate pelvic floor exercises into your daily routine, such as during brushing teeth, watching TV, or sitting at a desk.
    - **Progression:** Gradually increase the duration of each contraction and the

number of repetitions as your muscles become stronger.

'ips for Effective Pelvic Floor Exercises

1. **Avoid Overexertion:**
   - **Gentle Approach:** Start slowly and gradually increase the intensity. Overexerting the muscles can lead to fatigue and decreased effectiveness.

2. **Maintain Proper Breathing:**
   - **Breath Control:** Make sure you are breathing normally during the exercises. Not breathing can increase pressure in the abdomen and counter the effects of the exercises.

3. **Focus on Quality:**
   - **Proper Technique:** Ensure you are contracting the correct muscles. Avoid engaging the abdominal, buttock, or thigh muscles.

4. **Seek Professional Guidance:**
   - **Pelvic Floor Physiotherapy:** If you have difficulty identifying the pelvic floor muscles or are experiencing pelvic floor dysfunction, consider

consulting a pelvic floor physiotherapist for personalize guidance and support.

Pelvic floor exercises are a vital component o prenatal and postpartum care. By strengthening th pelvic floor muscles, expectant mothers car prepare their bodies for childbirth, reduce the risl of incontinence and prolapse, and enhance thei overall physical and mental well-being Postpartum, these exercises facilitate faste recovery, continued pelvic health, and improvec sexual function. Incorporating pelvic floor exercises into daily routines can yield long-term benefits, ensuring a healthier and more comfortable pregnancy and postpartum experience.

86

PART 4: Labor and Delivery

Chapter 7 Early Signs of Labor: Identifying the signs that labor is beginning and when to go to the hospital or birthing center.

Stages of Labor: Detailing the three stages of labor and what to expect during each phase.

The final stages of pregnancy are often filled with a mix of anticipation and anxiety as expectant parents look forward to the arrival of their baby. Recognizing the early signs of labor is crucial for knowing when to head to the hospital or birthing center, ensuring both the mother and baby receive timely care. Understanding these signs can help alleviate some of the uncertainty and provide a sense of readiness as the big day approaches.

Early Signs of Labor

1. **Lightening (Dropping)**
   - **Description:** Lightening occurs when the baby moves down into the pelvis, preparing for birth. This often happens a few weeks before labor begins, especially for first-time mothers.
   - **Signs:** Increased pressure in the pelvis, easier breathing as the baby moves away from the lungs, but potentially more frequent urination due to the added pressure on the bladder.
2. **Effacement and Dilation**

- o **Effacement:** This is known as the thinning of the cervix. Measured in percentages, a cervix that is 100% effaced is completely thinned out.
- o **Dilation:** Dilation is the opening of the cervix, measured in centimeters from 0 to 10. Active labor typically begins when the cervix is about 3-4 centimeters dilated.

3. **Bloody Show**
   - o **Description:** The "bloody show" is a discharge of mucus tinged with blood from the cervix. This mucus plug protects the uterus from infection and is released as the cervix begins to dilate.
   - o **Signs:** A thick, pinkish, or blood-streaked discharge, which can occur days or hours before labor starts.

4. **Nesting Instinct**
   - o **Description:** Many women experience a burst of energy and a strong desire to prepare their home for

the baby's arrival, known as th nesting instinct.

- o **Signs:** Sudden urge to clean, organize and set up the nursery, ofte accompanied by feelings o excitement and urgency.

5. **Back Pain and Cramps**

- o **Description:** Lower back pain anc menstrual-like cramps can indicate that labor is approaching, especially i they are consistent and progressively intensifying.
- o **Signs:** Persistent dull ache in the lower back, rhythmic cramping tha may radiate to the lower abdomen and thighs.

6. **Diarrhea**

- o **Description:** Hormonal changes preparing the body for labor can cause the bowels to become more active, leading to loose stools or diarrhea.
- o **Signs:** Frequent, loose bowel movements not related to illness or diet changes.

7. **Regular Contractions**

- o **Description:** Unlike Braxton Hicks contractions, which are irregular and often painless, true labor contractions are regular, painful, and increase in frequency and intensity.
- o **Signs:** Contractions that last 30-70 seconds, occurring at regular intervals and becoming closer together over time.

8. **Water Breaking**
   - o **Description:** The rupture of the amniotic sac, commonly referred to as the water breaking, can occur as a gush or a steady trickle of fluid.
   - o **Signs:** Sudden release of clear or slightly tinged fluid from the vagina. It can be difficult to distinguish from urine, but amniotic fluid is usually odorless and continues to leak.

When to Go to the Hospital or Birthing Center

Determining the right time to go to the hospital or birthing center is crucial to ensure a safe and smooth labor process. Here are guidelines to help make that decision:

1. **Contractions:**
   - **5-1-1 Rule:** A general guideline is to head to the hospital when contractions are five minutes apart, lasting one minute each, for at least one hour.
   - **Intensity:** If contractions are strong enough that you cannot walk or talk through them, it's likely time to go to the hospital.
2. **Water Breaking:**
   - **Immediate Contact:** Contact your healthcare provider immediately if your water breaks. They will advise you based on factors such as the color of the fluid and your Group B Strep status.
   - **Labor Onset:** Labor often starts within 24 hours of water breaking. If it doesn't, you may need medical assistance to induce labor to prevent infection.
3. **Bleeding:**
   - **Heavy Bleeding:** While a small amount of bloody show is normal, heavy bleeding like a menstrual

period is a sign to go to the hospital immediately, as it could indicate complications such as placental abruption.

4. **Decreased Fetal Movement:**
   - **Monitoring:** If you notice a significant decrease in your baby's movements, contact your healthcare provider. They may instruct you to go to the hospital for monitoring.

5. **Intense Pain:**
   - **Severe Discomfort:** If you experience severe or unusual pain that doesn't seem related to contractions, it's important to seek medical attention immediately. This could indicate complications.

6. **Maternal Instinct:**
   - **Trust Your Instincts:** If you feel something is not right or if you're unsure, it's always better to err on the side of caution and go to the hospital. Trust your instincts and don't hesitate to seek help.

Preparing for the Hospital or Birthing Center

Being prepared can reduce stress and ensure a smoother transition to the hospital or birthing center. Here are some tips:

1. **Hospital Bag:**
   - **Pack Early:** Have your hospital bag packed by 36 weeks. Include essentials such as comfortable clothing, toiletries, baby clothes, important documents, and any items that will make your stay more comfortable.
2. **Birth Plan:**
   - **Communicate Preferences:** Have a written birth plan outlining your preferences for labor, delivery, and postpartum care. Share this with your healthcare provider in advance and bring a copy to the hospital.
3. **Transportation:**
   - **Plan Ahead:** Ensure you have reliable transportation to the hospital or birthing center. Have a backup plan

in case your primary mode of transportation isn't available.

4. **Childcare:**
   - ○ **Arrange Childcare:** If you have other children, make arrangements for their care well in advance. Have a list of people you can call on short notice.

5. **Support System:**
   - ○ **Inform Your Support Team:** Keep your birth partner, family, and friends informed about your progress and when you're heading to the hospital. Having a support system in place can provide emotional and practical assistance.

Recognizing the early signs of labor and knowing when to go to the hospital or birthing center can help ensure a smoother, safer birth experience. Familiarizing yourself with these signs and having a plan in place can provide peace of mind as you approach the final stages of pregnancy. Trusting your body and staying in close communication with your healthcare provider will help you

navigate this exciting time with confidence an
readiness.

CONCLUSION

As you reach the end of "Pregnancy book for first time moms," it is my hope that you feel more empowered, informed, and prepared for the incredible journey that lies ahead. Pregnancy and childbirth are profound experiences that bring with them a unique blend of challenges and joys. By arming yourself with knowledge and practical strategies, you can navigate these experiences with greater confidence and ease.

Throughout this book, we have explored essential aspects of pregnancy and childbirth, from understanding the physical and emotional changes that occur during pregnancy to preparing your body for labour and ensuring a smooth postpartum recovery. We've delved into the importance of a balanced diet, the benefits of regular exercise, and the significance of pelvic floor health. We've also addressed specific conditions and provided guidance on how to manage them effectively.

The journey to motherhood is deeply personal and transformative. Each woman's experience is unique, and there is no one-size-fits-all approach. However, by embracing the principles and practices outlined in this guide, you can create a foundation of health and well-being that supports both you and your baby.

As you prepare for childbirth, remember to listen to your body and trust your instincts. Surround yourself with a supportive network of healthcare providers, family, and friends who can offer guidance and encouragement. And most importantly, be kind to yourself. Pregnancy and childbirth are demanding, and it's essential to acknowledge your strength and resilience every step of the way.

This book is just the beginning of your journey. Continue to seek out information, ask questions, and advocate for your needs. Your commitment to understanding and preparing for childbirth is a testament to your dedication as a mother. As you move forward, know that you have the tools and knowledge to face the challenges ahead with confidence and grace.

Wishing you a healthy, joyful, and empowering childbirth experience, and a wonderful beginning to motherhood. Here's to a beautiful, easy childbirth and a bright future with your new baby.